I0774446

WEIGHT LOSS

SECRETS REVEALED

A Practical Guide

S.O. AYOOLA

Copyright © 2024 S.O. AYOOLA

All rights reserved. No part of this publication may be reproduced, distributed, or transmitted in any form or by any means, including photocopying, recording, or other electronic or mechanical methods, without the prior written permission of the publisher, except in the case of brief quotations embodied in critical reviews and certain other noncommercial uses permitted by copyright law.

TABLE OF CONTENTS

I
INTRODUCTION

Starting a weight loss journey involves making changes in your life to become healthier. It's not just about shedding pounds; it's about embracing a lifestyle that supports your well-being. Practical approaches are essential, focusing on what works in the real world.

The journey is unique for everyone, with diverse motivations and goals. Some may seek weight loss for health reasons, while others aim for increased confidence or improved overall fitness. Regardless of the reasons, the key lies in adopting realistic and sustainable strategies.

Practicality is crucial in this context. It's not about extreme diets or intense workout regimens that are difficult to maintain. Instead, it's about finding a balance that fits into your daily life. Incorporating manageable changes ensures that the weight loss journey is not only effective but also enjoyable.

Understanding that there's no one-size-fits-all approach is pivotal. Genetics and lifestyle play significant roles in weight management. While some individuals may naturally have a higher metabolism, others may need to be more mindful of their choices. Recognizing these differences allows for personalized and effective strategies.

The importance of practicality extends to the methods chosen for weight loss. Rather than focusing on quick fixes, the emphasis should be on long-term habits. Crash diets may yield rapid results, but they often lead to unsustainable outcomes. Practical approaches involve making gradual and lasting changes to promote a healthier lifestyle.

In conclusion, the introduction sets the tone for a weight loss journey centered on practicality. It highlights the significance of realistic goals, sustainable plans, and an understanding of individual differences. The journey is not just about shedding pounds but embracing a healthier and more balanced way of living.

II

UNDERSTANDING WEIGHT LOSS

Weight loss is a complex process influenced by various factors, and understanding its intricacies is essential for anyone embarking on a journey towards a healthier lifestyle. At its core, weight loss is about achieving a balance between the calories you consume and the calories your body uses.

Calories play a pivotal role in weight management. They are units of energy found in the food and drinks we consume. To lose weight, you need to create a calorie deficit, meaning you burn more calories than you take in. This can be achieved through a combination of dietary changes and increased physical activity.

Metabolism, often used as a buzzword in the context of weight loss, refers to the processes your body undergoes to convert food and drink into energy. Basal metabolic rate (BMR) is the amount of energy your body needs at rest to maintain basic bodily functions, such as breathing and cell production. Understanding your BMR helps in determining the number of calories your body requires to function, which is crucial information for effective weight management.

Genetics can also play a significant role in how our bodies store and burn fat. Some individuals may have a genetic predisposition to be naturally lean, while others may be more prone to storing excess fat. While genetics can influence weight, lifestyle factors such as diet and physical activity remain powerful contributors.

Lifestyle choices have a profound impact on weight loss. Engaging in regular physical activity not only burns calories but also boosts metabolism and supports overall well-being. Sedentary habits, on the other hand, can contribute to weight gain. Finding a balance between diet and exercise is key to achieving and maintaining a healthy weight.

Setting realistic expectations is crucial when understanding weight loss. While some individuals may experience rapid initial results, progress tends to vary. It's essential to focus on overall health improvements rather than solely on the number on the scale. Sustainable weight loss takes time and involves adopting habits that can be maintained in the long run.

In conclusion, understanding weight loss involves grasping the basics of calories and metabolism, acknowledging the role of genetics, and recognizing the impact of lifestyle choices. It's a holistic approach that goes beyond the numbers, emphasizing a balanced and sustainable lifestyle for long-term success in achieving and maintaining a healthy weight.

III

SETTING REALISTIC GOALS

Setting realistic goals is a fundamental aspect of any successful weight loss journey. The acronym SMART - Specific, Measurable, Achievable, Relevant, and Time-bound - provides a framework for establishing effective objectives.

Specific goals define precisely what you want to achieve. Instead of a vague aim like "lose weight," a specific goal would be "lose 10 pounds in the next two months." Clarity in your objectives allows for a focused and purposeful approach to your weight loss journey.

Measurable goals involve tangible criteria to track your progress. Using the example above, the measure is the number of pounds lost. This quantifiable aspect not only helps in monitoring your success but also provides motivation as you witness tangible advancements.

Achievable goals ensure that your objectives are realistic and feasible. While aiming high is commendable, setting unattainable targets can lead to frustration and disappointment. Considering your current lifestyle, commitments, and capabilities is crucial when determining what is achievable for you.

Relevant goals align with your overall objectives. They should contribute directly to your weight loss journey. For instance, setting a goal to reduce sugar intake aligns with weight loss, while an unrelated goal might not yield the desired results.

Time-bound goals have a set timeframe for achievement. This adds a sense of urgency and helps prevent procrastination. Returning to the previous example, the goal of losing 10 pounds in the next two months provides a clear timeframe, pushing you to work consistently towards your target.

Creating a sustainable plan is another vital aspect of setting realistic goals. It involves establishing habits that can be maintained in the long term. Rapid and extreme changes may yield short-term results but are often difficult to sustain. A gradual approach, integrating healthier choices into your routine, ensures long-lasting success.

Balancing your goals across different aspects of your life is crucial. Weight loss is not solely about diet and exercise; it involves holistic lifestyle changes. Consider how your goals align with your work, family, and social life to ensure a well-rounded approach.

Support and accountability play integral roles in goal-setting. Sharing your objectives with friends, family, or a support group creates a network that can motivate and encourage you. Accountability keeps you on track, making it more likely that you'll stick to your goals.

In conclusion, setting realistic goals involves adopting the SMART criteria, ensuring specificity, measurability, achievability, relevance, and time-bound aspects. A sustainable plan, consideration of various life aspects, and the support of a network contribute to successful goal-setting in the context of a weight loss journey.

IV
NUTRITION ESSENTIALS

Nutrition is a cornerstone of any successful weight loss journey, and understanding the essentials is paramount for achieving and maintaining a healthy weight. Balanced diet principles form the foundation of effective nutrition strategies.

A balanced diet encompasses a variety of foods from different food groups, providing essential nutrients such as carbohydrates, proteins, fats, vitamins, and minerals. Striking the right balance ensures that your body receives the nutrients it needs for optimal functioning. Avoiding extreme diets and embracing a diverse range of foods is key to sustainable weight loss.

Portion control is a critical component of nutrition essentials. Even healthy foods can contribute to weight gain if consumed in excessive amounts. Understanding appropriate portion sizes helps in managing caloric intake and promotes mindful eating. This, in turn, supports weight loss by preventing overeating.

The importance of incorporating whole, unprocessed foods into your diet cannot be overstated. Whole foods, such as fruits, vegetables, whole grains, and lean proteins, are rich in nutrients and generally lower in calories than processed alternatives. Choosing these nutrient-dense options supports weight loss while ensuring your body receives essential vitamins and minerals.

Avoiding or moderating the intake of highly processed and sugary foods is crucial for weight management. Processed foods often contain added sugars, unhealthy fats, and excessive calories, contributing to weight gain. Opting for whole, minimally processed alternatives is a healthier choice.

Understanding the role of macronutrients is essential for effective weight loss. Carbohydrates, proteins, and fats are the primary macronutrients that provide energy and support various bodily functions. Striking a balance that suits your individual needs and goals is crucial. For instance, a moderate and balanced intake of healthy fats is essential for overall health and can contribute to satiety.

Hydration is often overlooked but plays a vital role in weight loss. Drinking an adequate amount of water helps control hunger, supports metabolism, and can prevent overeating. It's a simple yet powerful tool that should not be underestimated in the context of nutrition essentials.

Meal timing is another factor that can influence weight loss. While there's no one-size-fits-all approach, spreading meals throughout the day and avoiding large, infrequent meals can help regulate blood sugar levels, control hunger, and support weight loss efforts.

Educating yourself about nutritional labels is empowering. Understanding the information provided on food labels enables you to make informed choices about the products you consume. Paying attention to serving sizes, calories, and nutritional content assists in aligning your diet with your weight loss goals.

In conclusion, nutrition essentials for weight loss involve embracing a balanced diet, practicing portion control, choosing whole and minimally processed foods, moderating the intake of sugary and processed options, understanding macronutrients, prioritizing hydration, considering meal timing, and educating yourself about nutritional labels. These principles collectively contribute to a holistic and effective approach to nutrition in the context of a weight loss journey.

V

EFFECTIVE EXERCISE ROUTINES

Effective exercise routines are integral to a successful weight loss journey, contributing not only to the shedding of pounds but also to overall health and well-being. Simple and practical workouts that can be easily incorporated into daily life form the basis of these routines.

The concept of effective exercise goes beyond the traditional view of intense, time-consuming workouts. While high-intensity exercise has its benefits, incorporating manageable and enjoyable physical activity on a regular basis is key to long-term success.

Practicality is a cornerstone of effective exercise routines. Finding activities that fit into your lifestyle ensures consistency, a crucial factor in achieving and maintaining weight loss. This could include brisk walking, cycling, swimming, or any activity that gets your heart rate up and muscles working.

The importance of incorporating physical activity into daily life cannot be overstated. Rather than viewing exercise as a separate entity, integrating it into your routine makes it more sustainable. Simple changes like taking the stairs instead of the elevator, walking instead of driving for short distances, or engaging in quick home workouts can make a significant impact over time.

Strength training is a valuable component of effective exercise routines. Building muscle not only enhances your overall physique but also boosts metabolism. This means your body continues to burn calories even at rest, contributing to weight loss. Incorporating resistance exercises, whether using weights or your body weight, helps build and maintain muscle mass.

Cardiovascular exercises are essential for burning calories and improving heart health. Activities like running, jogging, cycling, or dancing elevate your heart rate, aiding in weight loss. These exercises also contribute to increased endurance and overall fitness.

Variety is key to keeping exercise routines interesting and preventing boredom. Trying different activities not only targets different muscle groups but also keeps you engaged. This could involve mixing up your workout routine with a combination of aerobic exercises, strength training, and flexibility exercises like yoga or pilates.

Consistency is paramount in any effective exercise routine. Rather than focusing on sporadic intense workouts, incorporating regular, moderate physical activity yields more sustainable results. Consistency builds habits, making it more likely for exercise to become a natural part of your routine.

Tailoring your exercise routine to your individual preferences is essential. Whether you enjoy outdoor activities, group classes, or home workouts, finding what you love ensures that you're more likely to stick with it. This personalization not only makes exercise more enjoyable but also increases the likelihood of long-term adherence.

Understanding your body's limits and gradually increasing intensity is crucial. Pushing yourself too hard too quickly can lead to burnout or injury. Gradually progressing in terms of duration, intensity, or complexity allows your body to adapt and reduces the risk of overexertion.

Incorporating flexibility exercises, such as stretching or yoga, promotes overall mobility and reduces the risk of injury. Flexibility is often overlooked but is essential for maintaining a healthy range of motion in joints and muscles.

In conclusion, effective exercise routines for weight loss involve practical, consistent, and enjoyable physical activity. Incorporating both cardiovascular and strength training exercises, maintaining variety, personalizing your routine, and understanding your body's limits are key elements. By viewing exercise as an integral part of daily life and embracing a holistic approach, you create a sustainable foundation for achieving and maintaining weight loss.

VI
MINDFUL EATING

Mindful eating is a powerful approach that goes beyond the traditional focus on what you eat, emphasizing how you eat and your relationship with food. Building awareness of eating habits and developing strategies for overcoming emotional eating are key components of mindful eating, contributing to a more balanced and sustainable approach to weight loss.

Building awareness of eating habits involves paying attention to the sensory aspects of food and the eating experience. This includes tuning into the taste, texture, and smell of food, as well as recognizing hunger and fullness cues. Mindful eating encourages being present in the moment, savoring each bite, and appreciating the nourishment food provides.

One fundamental aspect of mindful eating is recognizing and responding to hunger and fullness signals. Many individuals struggle with emotional or external triggers that lead to eating when not hungry or continuing to eat past the point of fullness. Mindful eating encourages listening to your body's natural cues, distinguishing between physical hunger and emotional cravings.

Developing a healthy relationship with food involves understanding the difference between physical and emotional hunger. Physical hunger arises gradually and is typically satisfied with a variety of foods, while emotional hunger tends to be sudden, specific, and often associated with particular cravings. Mindful eating helps in identifying these patterns and responding appropriately.

Emotional eating is a common challenge, often used as a coping mechanism for stress, boredom, or other emotions. Mindful eating strategies include finding alternative ways to cope with emotions, such as practicing deep breathing, going for a walk, or engaging in a favorite hobby.

Recognizing emotional triggers allows for more conscious and intentional choices.

Creating a mindful eating environment is another crucial aspect. This involves minimizing distractions, such as watching TV or working while eating, and focusing on the meal. Eating slowly and chewing food thoroughly not only aids digestion but also allows time for the brain to register feelings of fullness.

Practicing portion control is intertwined with mindful eating. Being mindful of portion sizes helps prevent overeating and allows for a more conscious evaluation of hunger and fullness cues. This approach promotes a healthier relationship with food and contributes to effective weight management.

The concept of mindful eating extends beyond individual meals to the overall eating experience. This involves considering the quality of the food you consume, opting for nutrient-dense options, and appreciating the impact of food choices on your well-being. Mindful eating encourages a non-restrictive, flexible approach that emphasizes nourishment rather than strict rules.

Strategies for overcoming emotional eating include keeping a food journal to track emotions associated with eating, seeking support from friends or a counselor, and practicing mindfulness techniques. Mindful breathing, meditation, or yoga can help manage stress and emotional triggers, fostering a more balanced relationship with food.

Incorporating mindful eating into social situations is essential. This involves being present during meals with others, engaging in conversation, and savoring the social aspect of sharing food. This approach encourages a positive and enjoyable relationship with meals, emphasizing the communal and cultural aspects of eating.

In conclusion, mindful eating is a holistic approach that emphasizes awareness of eating habits, recognition of hunger and fullness cues, and strategies for overcoming emotional eating. Building a healthy relationship with food involves being present in the eating experience, practicing portion control, and creating a mindful eating environment. By incorporating mindfulness into meals, individuals can foster a more balanced and sustainable approach to weight loss.

VII
SLEEP AND STRESS MANAGEMENT

Sleep and stress management are crucial components of a holistic approach to weight loss and overall well-being. Both factors play interconnected roles, influencing each other and impacting various aspects of health. Understanding the impact of sleep and stress on weight loss and adopting practical tips for better sleep and stress reduction are essential for achieving long-term success.

Sleep and Its Impact on Weight Loss:

Sleep is a fundamental aspect of health that often goes overlooked in the context of weight loss. Lack of adequate sleep can disrupt hormonal balance, affecting appetite regulation and metabolism. Two key hormones, ghrelin, and leptin, play pivotal roles in hunger and fullness signals.

Ghrelin, known as the hunger hormone, increases with insufficient sleep, promoting appetite and potentially leading to overeating. On the other hand, leptin, the hormone responsible for signaling fullness, decreases. This hormonal imbalance creates a situation where individuals may feel hungrier and less satisfied, contributing to potential weight gain.

In addition to hormonal influences, lack of sleep affects decision-making and impulse control. Fatigue can lead to poor food choices, increased cravings for high-calorie, sugary foods, and decreased motivation for physical activity. The cumulative impact of these factors can hinder weight loss efforts and make it challenging to maintain a healthy lifestyle.

Practical Tips for Better Sleep:

1. Establish a Consistent Sleep Schedule: Going to bed and waking up at the same time each day helps regulate your body's internal clock, promoting better sleep.

2. Create a Relaxing Bedtime Routine: Engage in calming activities before bedtime, such as reading, taking a warm bath, or practicing relaxation exercises.

3. Optimize Your Sleep Environment: Ensure your bedroom is conducive to sleep by keeping it dark, quiet, and cool. Invest in a comfortable mattress and pillows.

4. Limit Screen Time Before Bed: Exposure to blue light from screens can interfere with melatonin production, making it harder to fall asleep. Avoid screens at least an hour before bedtime.

5. Watch Your Diet: Avoid heavy meals, caffeine, and alcohol close to bedtime. These can disrupt sleep patterns and affect the quality of your rest.

Stress and Its Impact on Weight Loss:

Stress is a natural response to challenges, but chronic stress can have detrimental effects on both mental and physical health. In the context of weight loss, stress can lead to emotional eating, cravings for unhealthy foods, and the accumulation of abdominal fat.

Cortisol, often referred to as the stress hormone, plays a central role in the body's stress response. Elevated cortisol levels, especially when chronic, can lead to increased appetite and a preference for high-calorie foods. This physiological response is believed to be a survival mechanism, preparing the body to face potential threats.

Chronic stress can also disrupt sleep patterns, creating a vicious cycle. Poor sleep contributes to increased stress levels, and elevated stress levels can further hinder the ability to achieve restful sleep. Breaking this cycle is essential for overall well-being and effective weight management.

Practical Tips for Stress Reduction:

1. Incorporate Relaxation Techniques: Practices such as deep breathing, meditation, and progressive muscle relaxation can help manage stress levels.

2. Stay Active: Regular physical activity is a powerful stress reducer. Find activities you enjoy, whether it's walking, yoga, or dancing.

3. Establish Boundaries: Learn to say no and prioritize self-care. Setting realistic expectations and boundaries can help manage stress at work and in personal relationships.

4. Connect with Others: Social support is a crucial buffer against stress. Share your feelings with friends, family, or a support group.

5. Practice Time Management: Break tasks into smaller, manageable steps. Prioritize tasks and focus on what you can control.

The Interconnection of Sleep and Stress:

Recognizing the interconnection between sleep and stress is essential for a comprehensive approach to well-being. Stress can lead to sleep disturbances, and lack of sleep can exacerbate stress levels. Breaking this cycle involves addressing both factors simultaneously.

Creating a Holistic Approach:

1. Establish Healthy Habits: Adopting a routine that prioritizes both sleep and stress management is crucial. Consistency in bedtime, wake-up time, and stress reduction practices creates a stable foundation for well-being.

2. Mindfulness and Mind-Body Practices: Practices such as mindfulness meditation, yoga, and tai chi integrate both stress reduction and relaxation techniques. These holistic approaches contribute to improved sleep quality and reduced stress levels.

Conclusion:

In conclusion, sleep and stress management are integral aspects of a holistic approach to weight loss and overall health. Adequate sleep supports hormonal balance, appetite regulation, and decision-making, while effective stress management reduces the risk of emotional eating and promotes a healthier relationship with food.

Practical tips for better sleep and stress reduction involve establishing consistent routines, creating a conducive sleep environment, incorporating relaxation techniques, staying physically active, and fostering social connections. Recognizing the interconnection between sleep and stress allows for a more comprehensive and effective strategy in achieving and maintaining a healthy weight and well-being.

VIII

HYDRATION AND ITS ROLE

Hydration is a fundamental aspect of overall health and plays a crucial role in weight loss. Understanding the importance of water intake, recognizing signs of dehydration, and adopting practical ways to stay hydrated contribute to a well-rounded approach to well-being.

The Importance of Hydration:

Water is essential for the proper functioning of every cell, tissue, and organ in the body. It plays a vital role in various physiological processes, including digestion, nutrient absorption, temperature regulation, and waste elimination. Staying adequately hydrated is fundamental to maintaining optimal health and supporting the body's natural functions.

In the context of weight loss, hydration can be a valuable ally. Drinking water before meals can create a feeling of fullness, potentially reducing overall caloric intake. Choosing water over sugary beverages helps manage calorie consumption, contributing to weight loss efforts. Additionally, staying hydrated supports physical activity, enhancing exercise performance and aiding in the burning of calories.

Determining Hydration Needs:

Individual hydration needs vary based on factors such as age, sex, weight, activity level, and climate. The "8x8 rule," suggesting eight 8-ounce glasses of water a day, is a general guideline. However, specific hydration requirements may differ.

Listening to your body is crucial in determining hydration needs. Thirst is a natural indicator that your body requires water. Dark yellow urine can be a sign of dehydration, while light yellow or pale straw-colored urine is an indication of adequate hydration.

Factors such as physical activity, climate, and certain medical conditions can increase fluid requirements. Engaging in strenuous exercise, exposure to hot weather, or experiencing illness may necessitate increased water intake. Pregnant or breastfeeding individuals also have elevated hydration needs.

Practical Ways to Stay Hydrated:

1. Regular Water Intake: Drinking water throughout the day is the most straightforward method of staying hydrated. Keeping a water bottle with you and taking sips regularly helps meet your fluid requirements.

2. Hydrating Foods: Consuming foods with high water content, such as fruits and vegetables (e.g., watermelon, cucumber, and oranges), contributes to overall hydration.

3. Herbal Teas and Infusions: Unsweetened herbal teas and infusions provide a flavorful alternative to plain water. They can be enjoyed hot or cold, adding variety to your hydration routine.

4. Electrolyte Balance: Maintaining a balance of electrolytes, including sodium, potassium, and magnesium, is essential for hydration. Consuming electrolyte-rich foods and beverages, such as coconut water or sports drinks in moderation, helps support hydration.

5. Monitor Caffeine and Alcohol Intake: Caffeine and alcohol can have diuretic effects, increasing urine production and potentially leading to dehydration. Moderating intake and ensuring adequate water consumption counterbalances these effects.

6. Hydration Tracking Apps: Using mobile apps to track water intake can be a helpful tool. These apps often provide reminders to drink water regularly and help ensure that you meet your hydration goals.

7. Flavored Water: Adding natural flavors to water, such as a splash of lemon or cucumber, can make it more appealing. This can be a refreshing way to enhance water consumption.

8. Set Hydration Goals: Establishing daily hydration goals based on your individual needs provides a clear target. It can serve as a motivational tool to ensure consistent water intake.

Dehydration and Its Effects:

Dehydration occurs when the body loses more fluid than it takes in, leading to an imbalance in electrolytes and potential disruptions in bodily functions. Mild dehydration can result in symptoms such as thirst, dark urine, dry skin, and fatigue. Severe dehydration requires prompt medical attention and may present with symptoms like rapid heartbeat, sunken eyes, confusion, and dizziness.

Chronic dehydration can have long-term health implications, affecting kidney function, joint health, and overall well-being. In the context of weight loss, dehydration can be misleading. While initial weight loss may occur due to water loss, it is not a sustainable or healthy method for shedding pounds. Rehydrating is essential to restore normal bodily functions and support long-term health.

Hydration and Exercise:

Physical activity increases fluid requirements, and maintaining proper hydration is essential for exercise performance and recovery. Dehydration during exercise can lead to fatigue, decreased endurance, and an increased risk of heat-related illnesses.

Guidelines for hydration during exercise include:

- **Pre-exercise Hydration:** Drink water before starting your workout to ensure adequate fluid levels.

- **During Exercise:** Sip water throughout your workout, especially during intense or prolonged activities. The American Council on Exercise recommends consuming 7-10 ounces of water every 10-20 minutes during exercise.

- **Post-exercise Hydration:** Rehydrate after exercise by drinking water to replace fluids lost during the workout. Consuming a beverage with electrolytes can be beneficial, especially after intense or prolonged exercise.

Hydration and Weight Loss Plateaus:

Staying hydrated is a factor that is sometimes overlooked when facing weight loss plateaus. Dehydration can lead to water retention, masking true fat loss on the scale. Adequate water intake helps flush out excess sodium and waste products, reducing bloating and promoting a more accurate representation of weight loss progress.

Additionally, drinking water before meals can create a sense of fullness, potentially reducing overall calorie intake. This simple strategy aligns with mindful eating practices and supports weight loss efforts.

Conclusion:

In conclusion, hydration is a fundamental aspect of overall health and plays a significant role in weight loss. Recognizing the importance of adequate water intake, understanding individual hydration needs, and adopting practical strategies for staying hydrated contribute to a comprehensive approach to well-being.

By listening to your body, incorporating a variety of hydrating foods and beverages, and monitoring factors that may increase fluid requirements, you can maintain optimal hydration levels. Staying hydrated supports physical activity, aids in weight loss efforts, and promotes overall health and vitality.

IX
SUPERFOODS AND NUTRITIONAL SUPPLEMENTS

Superfoods and nutritional supplements have gained widespread attention for their potential health benefits, and they play a role in many individuals' approaches to nutrition and well-being. Understanding the concepts of superfoods and supplements, exploring the potential advantages and limitations, and considering guidance on their safe and effective use contribute to a comprehensive perspective on nutrition.

Superfoods: A Holistic Approach to Nutrition:

Superfoods are nutrient-dense foods that are rich in vitamins, minerals, antioxidants, and other beneficial compounds. They are often associated with potential health benefits and are considered valuable additions to a well-rounded diet. Incorporating a variety of superfoods can contribute to overall nutrient intake, supporting various bodily functions and promoting well-being.

Examples of commonly recognized superfoods include:

1. Berries (e.g., blueberries, strawberries, and raspberries): Packed with antioxidants, vitamins, and fiber, berries are celebrated for their potential in promoting heart health and reducing inflammation.

2. Leafy Greens (e.g., kale, spinach, and Swiss chard): These greens are abundant in vitamins, minerals, and antioxidants, supporting immune function, bone health, and overall vitality.

3. Nuts and Seeds (e.g., almonds, chia seeds, and flaxseeds): Rich in healthy fats, protein, and fiber, nuts and seeds are associated with heart health and may aid in weight management.

4. Fatty Fish (e.g., salmon, mackerel, and sardines): High in omega-3 fatty acids, fatty fish are linked to cardiovascular health and cognitive function.

5. Turmeric: Known for its anti-inflammatory properties, turmeric contains the active compound curcumin, which has been studied for its potential health benefits.

6. Quinoa: A protein-rich grain alternative, quinoa provides essential amino acids and is a good source of fiber, vitamins, and minerals.

Advantages of Superfoods:

1. Rich in Nutrients: Superfoods are nutrient powerhouses, providing a concentrated source of vitamins, minerals, antioxidants, and other beneficial compounds.

2. Diverse Health Benefits: Many superfoods are associated with specific health benefits, such as improved heart health, reduced inflammation, and enhanced cognitive function.

3. Supportive of Overall Well-being: Incorporating a variety of superfoods into a balanced diet can contribute to overall health, supporting various bodily functions and promoting vitality.

Limitations and Considerations:

1. No Single "Magic Bullet": While superfoods offer valuable nutrients, there is no single food that can provide all the essential nutrients the body needs. A diverse and balanced diet is essential.

2. Nutrient Interaction: Some nutrients in superfoods may interact with medications or have contraindications for certain health conditions. It's crucial to consult with a healthcare professional if you have concerns or specific health considerations.

3. Accessibility and Affordability: Not all superfoods are readily available or affordable for everyone. It's essential to focus on a variety of nutrient-dense foods within one's budget and geographical availability.

Nutritional Supplements: Enhancing Dietary Intake:

Nutritional supplements encompass a wide range of products, including vitamins, minerals, amino acids, herbal extracts, and other substances. They are designed to complement dietary intake and address specific nutritional needs. While supplements can be beneficial in certain situations, their use should be guided by individual health goals, deficiencies, and consultation with healthcare professionals.

Common Types of Nutritional Supplements:

1. Multivitamins: Comprehensive supplements that typically contain a combination of vitamins and minerals to fill potential nutrient gaps in the diet.

2. Vitamin D: Especially important for bone health, vitamin D supplements may be recommended for individuals with limited sun exposure or specific health conditions.

3. Omega-3 Fatty Acids: Often derived from fish oil, omega-3 supplements provide essential fatty acids associated with heart health and cognitive function.

4. Calcium and Magnesium: Essential minerals for bone health, these supplements may be recommended for individuals with inadequate dietary intake.

5. Protein Supplements: Commonly used by athletes or those with increased protein needs, protein supplements come in various forms, including powders and bars.

6. Herbal Supplements: Extracts from plants or herbs, these supplements are often used for their potential health benefits, such as immune support or stress reduction.

Advantages of Nutritional Supplements:

1. Addressing Nutrient Deficiencies: Supplements can be valuable for individuals with specific nutrient deficiencies, helping restore optimal nutrient levels.

2. Convenience: Supplements provide a convenient way to obtain certain nutrients, especially for individuals with busy lifestyles or specific dietary restrictions.

3. Targeted Support: Certain supplements, such as omega-3 fatty acids or vitamin D, offer targeted support for specific health concerns.

Limitations and Considerations:

1. Not a Substitute for Whole Foods: Supplements should not replace a varied and balanced diet. Whole foods offer a complex matrix of nutrients, fiber, and other compounds that supplements may not replicate.

2. Potential for Overconsumption: Excessive intake of certain vitamins and minerals through supplements can have adverse effects. It's crucial to follow recommended dosage guidelines.

3. Quality and Safety Concerns: The supplement industry is not regulated as rigorously as pharmaceuticals, and the quality of products can vary. Choosing reputable brands and consulting healthcare professionals can help address safety concerns.

Guidance for Safe and Effective Use:

1. Consult with Healthcare Professionals: Before incorporating superfoods or nutritional supplements into your routine, consult with healthcare professionals, especially if you have underlying health conditions, are pregnant, or are taking medications.

2. Focus on a Balanced Diet: While superfoods and supplements can complement dietary intake, the foundation of nutrition should be a diverse and balanced diet that includes a variety of whole foods.

3. Individualized Approach: Consider individual health goals, nutritional needs, and potential deficiencies when deciding on the use of supplements. What works for one person may not be suitable for another.

4. Mindful Consumption: Use supplements mindfully, avoiding excessive intake. More is not always better, and following recommended dosage guidelines is crucial for safety.

5. Monitor for Adverse Effects: Pay attention to how your body responds to supplements. If you experience adverse effects or have concerns, seek guidance from healthcare professionals.

Conclusion:

In conclusion, superfoods and nutritional supplements can be valuable components of a holistic approach to nutrition, supporting overall well-being and addressing specific health needs. Understanding their advantages, limitations, and considerations is essential for making informed choices that align with individual health goals.

By incorporating a diverse range of nutrient-dense foods, focusing on a balanced diet, and using supplements judiciously with guidance from healthcare professionals, individuals can create a comprehensive and sustainable approach to nutrition that contributes to overall health and vitality.

X
SOCIAL SUPPORT AND ACCOUNTABILITY

Social support and accountability play pivotal roles in achieving and maintaining various goals, including those related to weight loss and overall well-being. Building a supportive environment and sharing goals with others create a network that fosters motivation, encouragement, and a sense of community. This comprehensive exploration delves into the significance of social support, the impact of accountability, and practical strategies for integrating them into one's journey.

The Power of Social Support:

Human beings are inherently social creatures, and the influence of our social connections extends to various aspects of life, including health and lifestyle choices. Social support refers to the assistance, encouragement, and understanding received from others. In the context of weight loss and well-being, social support provides a foundation for motivation, resilience, and sustained effort.

Types of Social Support:

1. Emotional Support: This involves expressing care, empathy, and understanding. Emotional support is crucial during challenging times and can provide a sense of belonging and connection.

2. Instrumental Support: Practical assistance or tangible aid falls under instrumental support. This can include help with meal preparation, exercise routines, or any actions that contribute directly to health goals.

3. Informational Support: Providing information, advice, or guidance is informational support. This can be valuable in navigating dietary choices, exercise routines, or understanding health-related information.

4. Appraisal Support: Constructive feedback and positive reinforcement constitute appraisal support. Having others acknowledge and celebrate achievements contributes to motivation.

Benefits of Social Support:

1. Motivation and Accountability: Knowing that others are invested in your goals provides a motivational boost. The sense of accountability to friends, family, or a community encourages consistent effort.

2. Stress Reduction: Sharing concerns and challenges with a supportive network can alleviate stress. Emotional support helps in coping with difficulties and maintaining focus on health goals.

3. Behavioral Modeling: Observing and participating in healthy behaviors within a social circle promotes positive habits. Shared experiences create a culture of wellness.

4. Increased Likelihood of Success: Research consistently shows that individuals with strong social support are more likely to achieve and maintain their health and weight loss goals.

Building a Supportive Environment:

1. Communicate Openly: Share your health goals, challenges, and achievements with those close to you. Open communication fosters understanding and allows others to provide effective support.

2. Choose Supportive Relationships: Surround yourself with individuals who encourage your well-being and share similar health goals. Positive influences contribute to a supportive environment.

3. Join Communities: Engaging in groups or communities focused on health and wellness provides a sense of belonging. Online forums, local fitness classes, or support groups offer opportunities for connection.

4. Family Involvement: Incorporate family members into your health journey. Plan and prepare meals together, engage in physical activities as a family, and create a shared commitment to well-being.

The Role of Accountability:

Accountability is the obligation or willingness to accept responsibility for one's actions. In the context of health and weight loss, accountability serves as a powerful motivator, promoting consistency and adherence to established goals.

Forms of Accountability:

1. Self-Accountability: Setting personal goals, tracking progress, and holding oneself responsible for actions fall under self-accountability. This involves intrinsic motivation and discipline.

2. External Accountability: External sources, such as friends, family, or a mentor, can provide accountability. Sharing goals with others and providing regular updates create external structures for responsibility.

Benefits of Accountability:

1. Consistency: Knowing that others are aware of your goals encourages consistent effort. Regular check-ins and updates contribute to a routine of healthy behaviors.

2. Goal Clarity: Accountability prompts individuals to define and clarify their goals. This specificity increases the likelihood of success by providing clear targets.

3. Adaptability: Regular accountability check-ins allow for adjustments to goals and strategies. This adaptability is crucial in navigating challenges and refining approaches based on progress and setbacks.

4. Momentum: Consistent accountability builds momentum. Small, regular achievements contribute to a sense of accomplishment and reinforce positive behaviors.

Practical Strategies for Social Support and Accountability:

1. Share Your Goals: Communicate your health and weight loss goals with friends, family, or a supportive community. Sharing goals creates a sense of commitment and invites encouragement.

2. Create Accountability Partnerships: Pairing up with a friend or family member for mutual support and accountability is effective. Regular check-ins and shared progress contribute to a collaborative effort.

3. Join Fitness Classes or Groups: Participating in fitness classes or groups not only provides an opportunity for regular physical activity but also creates a supportive community with shared goals.

4. Utilize Technology: Fitness apps, social media groups, or online forums dedicated to health and wellness offer virtual communities for support and accountability.

5. Engage in Group Challenges: Organize or participate in group challenges that align with health goals. These challenges create a collective commitment and foster a sense of camaraderie.

6. Regular Check-Ins: Establish a routine for regular check-ins with accountability partners. This can be weekly or bi-weekly meetings to discuss progress, challenges, and adjustments to goals.

7. Celebrate Achievements: Acknowledge and celebrate both small and significant achievements. Positive reinforcement enhances motivation and strengthens the commitment to health goals.

8. Create Shared Activities: Incorporate shared physical activities into social gatherings. This can include hiking, cycling, or participating in sports, making well-being a collective focus.

9. Seek Professional Support: Consider involving healthcare professionals, nutritionists, or personal trainers in your health journey. Their expertise adds an additional layer of accountability and guidance.

Overcoming Challenges:

1. Resistance to Change: Some individuals may resist changes in lifestyle habits. Encourage open communication, share information on the benefits of health improvements, and focus on gradual, sustainable changes.

2. Negative Influences: Addressing negative influences requires clear communication about personal goals and boundaries. Surrounding oneself with positive influences can counteract negativity.

3. Lack of Time: Prioritize health and well-being by scheduling dedicated time for physical activity and meal preparation. Communicate the importance of these commitments to those in your support network.

Conclusion:

In conclusion, social support and accountability are integral components of a successful journey towards health and weight loss. Building a supportive environment, sharing goals with others, and incorporating accountability structures create a foundation for motivation, consistency, and resilience.

By fostering open communication, choosing supportive relationships, and actively participating in communities focused on well-being, individuals can create a network that contributes to their overall health and success in achieving and maintaining their health goals. Integrating these principles into daily life enhances the journey towards well-being.

XI
OVERCOMING PLATEAUS AND CHALLENGES

Overcoming plateaus and challenges is a crucial aspect of any transformative journey, especially when pursuing weight loss or health goals. Plateaus, where progress seems to stall, and challenges, which are inevitable obstacles, require strategic approaches to navigate and continue moving forward. This comprehensive exploration delves into the nature of plateaus and challenges, the factors contributing to their occurrence, and practical strategies to overcome them.

Understanding Plateaus:

Plateaus are periods where progress in achieving weight loss or health goals slows down or halts altogether. They can be frustrating, demotivating, and lead to a sense of stagnation. Understanding the factors contributing to plateaus is key to devising effective strategies for overcoming them.

Factors Contributing to Plateaus:

1. Metabolic Adaptation: The body adapts to changes in diet and exercise, leading to a slowdown in metabolism. As the body becomes more efficient at utilizing energy, weight loss may plateau.

2. Caloric Intake vs. Expenditure: If the calories consumed match the calories expended, weight loss can plateau. Adjustments in diet and exercise may be necessary to break through.

3. Lack of Variety in Exercise: Performing the same exercises repeatedly can lead to a plateau as the body adapts. Incorporating variety challenges different muscle groups and can stimulate progress.

4. Inadequate Recovery: Insufficient rest and recovery can impede progress. The body needs time to repair and rebuild, especially after intense workouts.

5. Stress and Cortisol Levels: Elevated stress levels can lead to increased cortisol production, which may contribute to weight loss plateaus. Managing stress is crucial for overall well-being.

6. Hydration Levels: Inadequate hydration can impact metabolism and energy levels. Proper hydration is essential for various bodily functions, including those related to weight loss.

Strategies for Overcoming Plateaus:

1. Reevaluate and Adjust Goals: Periodically reassess your goals and expectations. Setting realistic and achievable targets helps maintain motivation and reduces frustration during plateaus.

2. Modify Exercise Routine: Introduce variety into your workout routine. Incorporate different types of exercises, change intensity levels, or explore new activities to challenge your body.

3. Review Nutrition Plan: Analyze your dietary habits. Ensure you are consuming a balanced and varied diet. Adjusting caloric intake based on changing needs can help overcome plateaus.

4. Strength Training: Incorporating strength training exercises builds muscle mass, which can boost metabolism. Muscle tissue burns more calories at rest than fat tissue.

5. Interval Training: High-intensity interval training (HIIT) alternates between short bursts of intense exercise and periods of rest. This approach can be effective in breaking through plateaus.

6. Adequate Sleep: Prioritize quality sleep as it plays a crucial role in overall health, metabolism, and recovery. Lack of sleep can contribute to stress and hinder weight loss efforts.

7. Hydration: Ensure proper hydration by drinking enough water throughout the day. Hydration supports metabolism, aids in digestion, and can contribute to increased energy levels.

Common Weight Loss Challenges:

Weight loss challenges are inevitable on any health journey. Identifying and understanding these challenges is the first step in developing effective strategies for overcoming them.

Common Weight Loss Challenges Include:

1. Emotional Eating: Using food as a coping mechanism for stress, boredom, or emotions can undermine weight loss efforts.

2. Cravings: Intense desires for specific foods, especially those high in sugar or unhealthy fats, can be challenging to resist.

3. Lack of Motivation: Maintaining consistent motivation over the long term can be difficult. External and internal factors can influence motivation levels.

4. Time Constraints: Balancing work, family, and other commitments may lead to challenges in finding time for regular exercise and meal preparation.

5. Social Pressures: Social situations, gatherings, or peer influences can pose challenges in sticking to a healthy eating plan.

6. Plateaus and Stalls: Periods where weight loss slows down or halts can be demotivating and may require adjustments to break through.

7. Injuries or Health Issues: Physical injuries or health conditions can limit exercise options and impact overall well-being.

Strategies for Overcoming Weight Loss Challenges:

1. Mindful Eating: Building awareness of eating habits and recognizing triggers for emotional eating can help in developing healthier responses to challenges.

2. Meal Planning: Plan and prepare meals in advance to avoid making unhealthy food choices due to time constraints or lack of options.

3. Seek Support: Share your challenges with friends, family, or a support network. Having a support system provides encouragement and understanding during difficult times.

4. Set Realistic Goals: Establish achievable and realistic short-term and long-term goals. Setting the bar too high can lead to frustration and loss of motivation.

5. Incorporate Physical Activity: Find enjoyable ways to stay active, even in time-constrained situations. Short bursts of activity throughout the day can add up.

6. Diversify Workouts: Engage in a variety of physical activities to prevent boredom and stimulate different muscle groups.

XII

CELEBRATING SUCCESS AND MAINTAINING PROGRESS

Celebrating success and maintaining progress are integral components of any transformative journey, especially when pursuing health and well-being goals. Recognizing achievements, whether big or small, provides motivation, reinforces positive behaviors, and contributes to sustained progress. This comprehensive exploration delves into the significance of celebrating success, the psychology behind rewards, and practical strategies for maintaining momentum and long-term progress.

The Significance of Celebrating Success:

Celebrating success is not merely an indulgence; it is a powerful psychological tool that reinforces positive behaviors and motivates continued effort. Acknowledging achievements, no matter how small, creates a positive feedback loop that fosters a sense of accomplishment, boosts self-esteem, and strengthens the commitment to one's goals.

Psychology Behind Rewards and Celebration:

Understanding the psychological mechanisms at play when celebrating success provides insights into why this practice is effective in maintaining progress:

1. Positive Reinforcement: Celebrating success acts as positive reinforcement for desired behaviors. When individuals associate their efforts with positive outcomes, they are more likely to repeat those behaviors.

2. Neurotransmitter Release: Success and celebration trigger the release of neurotransmitters like dopamine, often referred to as the "feel-good" neurotransmitter. This creates a sense of pleasure and reinforces the connection between effort and reward.

3. Behavioral Conditioning: Celebrating success contributes to behavioral conditioning. Over time, the brain forms associations between certain actions (efforts towards health goals) and the positive feelings experienced during celebrations.

4. Enhanced Motivation: Knowing that success will be acknowledged and celebrated enhances motivation. This anticipation acts as a driving force, encouraging individuals to persevere in their efforts.

Practical Strategies for Celebrating Success:

1. Set Milestones and Goals: Break down larger goals into smaller, achievable milestones. Celebrate these milestones to acknowledge progress and maintain motivation throughout the journey.

2. Personalized Rewards: Choose rewards that are meaningful and personally significant. This could be a treat, a relaxing activity, or anything that brings joy and satisfaction.

3. Share Achievements: Share your successes with friends, family, or a support network. Their positive reinforcement and acknowledgment amplify the sense of accomplishment.

4. Create a Success Journal: Keep a journal where you document your achievements, both big and small. Reflecting on past successes can serve as a source of motivation during challenging times.

5. Reward Jars or Charts: Create a visual representation of your progress using jars or charts. Each time you achieve a goal or milestone, add a token or mark to visually track your success.

6. Plan Celebration Events: Plan specific celebrations for reaching major milestones. This could be a special meal, a day out, or any event that feels like a reward for your hard work.

7. Incorporate Intrinsic Rewards: Find joy in the intrinsic rewards of your efforts. Feeling healthier, having more energy, or achieving a personal best in fitness are intrinsic rewards worth celebrating.

Maintaining Progress:

Maintaining progress is often more challenging than initiating change. It requires ongoing commitment, adaptability, and a mindset focused on long-term well-being. Here are practical strategies for sustaining progress:

1. Cultivate Healthy Habits: Shift the focus from short-term goals to cultivating sustainable, healthy habits. Consistent habits form the foundation for long-term success.

2. Set Realistic Expectations: Establish realistic expectations for the journey. Understand that progress may have fluctuations, and setbacks are natural. Embrace the process as part of the overall transformation.

3. Adapt to Changing Circumstances: Life is dynamic, and circumstances may change. Be adaptable and open to adjusting your approach to fit evolving situations while staying aligned with your goals.

4. Regular Check-Ins: Periodically assess your goals, habits, and progress. Regular check-ins help you stay on track, identify areas for improvement, and celebrate ongoing successes.

5. Establish a Support Network: Surround yourself with individuals who support your goals. Share your journey with friends, family, or a community that understands and encourages your commitment to well-being.

6. Mindful Eating Practices: Embrace mindful eating to foster a healthy relationship with food. Pay attention to hunger cues, savor each bite, and make conscious choices that align with your nutritional goals.

7. Diversify Physical Activities: Keep physical activities enjoyable by diversifying your routine. Explore different forms of exercise to prevent monotony and maintain enthusiasm for staying active.

8. Prioritize Sleep and Stress Management: Quality sleep and effective stress management are foundational to overall well-being. Prioritize both to ensure you have the energy and resilience needed for sustained progress.

9. Continual Learning: Stay informed and engaged in continual learning about nutrition, exercise, and overall health. Knowledge empowers you to make informed decisions that contribute to long-term well-being.

10. Celebrate Non-Scale Victories: Progress extends beyond the number on the scale. Celebrate non-scale victories such as increased energy levels, improved mood, enhanced fitness, or clothing fitting better.

Overcoming Setbacks:

Setbacks are a natural part of any transformative journey. How you respond to setbacks significantly influences your ability to maintain progress. Here are strategies for overcoming setbacks:

1. Reflect without Judgment: When facing a setback, reflect on the circumstances without self-judgment. Understand what led to the setback and use it as an opportunity for learning.

2. Adjust Goals if Necessary: If setbacks are recurrent, consider reassessing your goals. Adjusting goals to align with realistic expectations and current circumstances helps maintain motivation.

3. Seek Support: Share setbacks with your support network. Seek encouragement, advice, or simply a listening ear. Supportive relationships can help you navigate challenges more effectively.

4. Reframe Negative Thoughts: Reframe negative thoughts that may accompany setbacks. Instead of viewing a setback as a failure, see it as a temporary obstacle on the path to long-term success.

5. Implement Positive Changes: Use setbacks as a catalyst for positive changes. Identify areas where adjustments can be made, and implement changes that contribute to ongoing progress.

6. Practice Self-Compassion: Be kind to yourself during setbacks. Understand that everyone faces challenges, and setbacks do not define your overall journey. Treat yourself with the same compassion you would offer a friend.

XIII

FAQS AND TROUBLESHOOTING

Let's dive into a comprehensive exploration of frequently asked questions (FAQs) and troubleshooting common challenges related to weight loss and overall well-being.

Frequently Asked Questions (FAQs):

1. Q: What is the most effective way to lose weight?

A: The most effective way to lose weight involves a combination of healthy eating, regular physical activity, and lifestyle changes. It's essential to create a sustainable plan tailored to your individual needs, focusing on a balanced diet, portion control, and consistent exercise.

2. Q: Are fad diets effective for weight loss?

A: Fad diets may result in short-term weight loss, but they often lack sustainability and can be unhealthy. Long-term success is better achieved through a balanced and varied diet that provides essential nutrients. Consult a healthcare professional for personalized advice.

3. Q: How many calories should I consume to lose weight?

A: Caloric needs vary, but a general guideline is to create a calorie deficit by consuming fewer calories than you burn. A deficit of 500 calories per day can lead to about one pound of weight loss per week. However, individual factors such as metabolism and activity level should be considered.

4. Q: Is spot reduction possible for losing fat in specific areas?

A: Spot reduction, targeting fat loss in specific areas through exercises, is a myth. Fat loss occurs throughout the body, influenced by overall calorie expenditure. Focus on full-body exercises, strength training, and cardiovascular activities for holistic results.

5. Q: How important is hydration for weight loss?

A: Hydration is crucial for overall health and can support weight loss. Drinking water before meals may help control appetite, and staying hydrated aids in metabolism. Replace sugary beverages with water to reduce calorie intake.

6. Q: Can I eat carbs and still lose weight?

A: Yes, you can include carbohydrates in your diet while losing weight. Opt for whole grains, fruits, and vegetables for complex carbohydrates that provide essential nutrients and fiber. Monitor portion sizes and choose nutrient-dense sources.

7. Q: How does stress affect weight loss?

A: Chronic stress can influence weight loss negatively. Stress may lead to emotional eating, increased cortisol levels (linked to fat storage), and disrupted sleep. Incorporate stress-management techniques like meditation and exercise into your routine.

8. Q: What role does sleep play in weight loss?

A: Adequate sleep is crucial for weight loss. Poor sleep can disrupt hormonal balance, increasing hunger hormones and decreasing satiety hormones. Aim for 7-9 hours of quality sleep per night to support overall well-being.

9. Q: Should I skip meals to lose weight faster?

A: Skipping meals is not recommended. It can lead to overeating later in the day and may negatively impact metabolism. Focus on regular, balanced meals to maintain steady energy levels and support weight loss.

10. Q: How can I stay motivated during my weight loss journey?

A: Set realistic goals, celebrate achievements, and involve a support network. Find activities you enjoy, vary your routine, and focus on non-scale victories. Regularly reassess your goals to maintain motivation throughout the journey.

Troubleshooting Common Challenges:

1. Challenge: Plateau in Weight Loss Progress

Solution: Reevaluate your nutrition and exercise plan. Adjust caloric intake, introduce variety in workouts, and consider factors like stress and sleep. Small changes can reignite progress.

2. Challenge: Emotional Eating

Solution: Develop mindfulness around eating habits. Identify triggers, practice stress-management techniques, and find alternative coping mechanisms. Seek support if emotional eating persists.

3. Challenge: Time Constraints for Exercise

Solution: Prioritize physical activity by scheduling it into your routine. Incorporate short, intense workouts or break exercise into smaller sessions. Choose activities you enjoy to make it a sustainable part of your day.

4. Challenge: Social Pressures and Unhealthy Eating Habits

Solution: Communicate your health goals with friends and family. Make healthier choices when dining out, and consider hosting gatherings with nutritious options. Build a supportive network that understands your commitment.

5. Challenge: Lack of Motivation

Solution: Reconnect with your goals, celebrate achievements, and visualize success. Find a workout buddy, join a class, or seek professional guidance for renewed motivation. Incorporate enjoyable activities into your routine.

6. Challenge: Injuries or Health Issues

Solution: Consult a healthcare professional before resuming exercise after an injury. Modify workouts to accommodate health conditions. Focus on nutrition and adapt activities to maintain overall well-being.

7. Challenge: Cravings for Unhealthy Foods

Solution: Identify triggers for cravings and replace unhealthy options with nutritious alternatives. Practice moderation, stay hydrated, and plan balanced meals to reduce cravings.

8. Challenge: Lack of Sleep

Solution: Prioritize sleep by establishing a consistent sleep routine. Create a sleep-friendly environment, limit screen time before bed, and manage stress to improve sleep quality.

9. Challenge: Balancing Work and Well-being

Solution: Schedule dedicated time for meal preparation and physical activity. Incorporate short bursts of exercise throughout the day. Delegate tasks when possible to create balance.

10. Challenge: Overcoming Setbacks

Solution: Reflect without judgment on setbacks, adjust goals if needed, and seek support. Use setbacks as opportunities for learning and implement positive changes. Practice self-compassion during challenging times.

In navigating FAQs and troubleshooting challenges, a personalized and adaptable approach is key. Consult with healthcare professionals when needed, stay connected with your support network, and celebrate both small victories and the overall progress on your health journey. Remember that each step forward, no matter how small, contributes to your long-term well-being.

XIV

INSPIRATIONAL STORIES

Let's explore a collection of inspirational stories that highlight the resilience, determination, and transformative journeys of individuals pursuing health and well-being. These stories showcase the diverse paths people have taken to overcome challenges, embrace positive changes, and achieve their goals.

Story 1: Sarah's Journey to a Healthier Lifestyle

Sarah, a busy professional, found herself caught in a cycle of stress, unhealthy eating, and sedentary habits. Realizing the impact on her well-being, she embarked on a journey to prioritize her health. Sarah started with small changes, incorporating short walks during breaks and opting for nutritious meals. Over time, she discovered a love for yoga, which not only improved her physical health but also became a powerful stress-management tool. Sarah's story emphasizes the importance of gradual changes, finding activities you enjoy, and the transformative impact of prioritizing self-care.

Story 2: John's Weight Loss Transformation

John's weight had been a source of insecurity and health concerns throughout his life. Determined to make a lasting change, he sought professional guidance and embraced a holistic approach to weight loss. John incorporated a balanced diet, regular exercise, and mindfulness practices into his routine. With perseverance and support from a community of like-minded individuals, he not only achieved his weight loss goal but also discovered a newfound confidence and passion for helping others on their health journeys.

Story 3: Maria's Triumph Over Emotional Eating

Maria's relationship with food was deeply intertwined with her emotions. Stress and emotional triggers led to unhealthy eating habits, hindering her weight loss efforts. Through self-reflection and support from a therapist, Maria addressed the root causes of her emotional eating. She learned healthier coping mechanisms and gradually redefined her relationship with food. Maria's story highlights the significance of addressing emotional well-being in the journey toward a healthier lifestyle.

Story 4: Mark's Fitness Renaissance in Midlife

Approaching midlife, Mark felt the need for a significant change. Despite a sedentary job and years of neglecting his fitness, he decided it was never too late to prioritize health. Mark started with simple exercises and gradually progressed to more challenging workouts. His journey was marked by perseverance, consistency, and a shift in mindset. Mark not only regained his physical fitness but also became an advocate for embracing a healthy lifestyle at any age.

Story 5: Emily's Transformation Through Mindful Eating

Emily's struggle with yo-yo dieting and self-esteem led her to explore mindful eating. She learned to savor each bite, listen to her body's hunger and fullness cues, and cultivate a positive relationship with food. Through mindful eating practices, Emily not only achieved sustainable weight loss but also developed a deeper appreciation for nourishing her body. Her story underscores the importance of tuning into one's body and fostering a mindful approach to nutrition.

Story 6: Jake's Fitness Journey from Couch to Marathon

Jake, a self-professed couch potato, decided to challenge himself by taking up running. Starting with short jogs, he gradually increased his distance and set a goal to complete a marathon. With consistent training, support from a running community, and a mindset of perseverance, Jake not only finished the marathon but transformed his sedentary lifestyle into an active one. His story is a testament to the transformative power of setting ambitious goals and taking gradual steps to achieve them.

Story 7: Lily's Resilience in Overcoming Health Challenges

Lily faced significant health challenges, including chronic illnesses that affected her mobility. Determined to improve her well-being, Lily focused on what she could control—her mindset and nutrition. She adapted her exercise routine to accommodate her health condition and prioritized nutrient-rich foods. Lily's resilience in the face of adversity exemplifies the impact of a positive mindset and making the best choices within one's unique circumstances.

Story 8: Carlos's Journey to Mental and Physical Strength

Carlos, a military veteran, struggled with post-traumatic stress disorder (PTSD) and associated challenges. Seeking a holistic approach to healing, he integrated physical fitness into his mental health journey. Regular exercise became a powerful tool for managing stress and improving Carlos's overall well-being. His story emphasizes the interconnectedness of mental and physical health, demonstrating how exercise can be a therapeutic outlet for those facing mental health challenges.

Story 9: Anna's Sustainable Approach to Wellness

Anna, a busy mother of three, embraced a sustainable approach to wellness that prioritized balance and self-compassion. She incorporated family-friendly activities like hiking and cooking nutritious meals together. Anna's story showcases the importance of finding a lifestyle that fits into

the demands of daily life, making health a family affair, and celebrating the journey as a collective achievement.

Story 10: David's Triumph Over Type 2 Diabetes

David's diagnosis of type 2 diabetes served as a wake-up call to prioritize his health. With guidance from healthcare professionals, he adopted a tailored nutrition plan and embraced regular exercise. Through consistent lifestyle changes, David not only managed his diabetes but also experienced significant improvements in overall health. His story highlights the transformative impact of lifestyle modifications in managing chronic conditions.

Conclusion:

These inspirational stories reflect the diversity of health journeys, the power of resilience, and the transformative impact of positive choices. Whether overcoming emotional eating, achieving weight loss goals, or embracing fitness at any age, these individuals showcase that sustainable change is possible with determination, support, and a commitment to overall well-being. Each story serves as a source of inspiration and encouragement for those on their own journeys toward a healthier and happier life.

XV
CONCLUSION

In conclusion, the journey toward health and well-being is a dynamic and individualized process, encompassing a multitude of factors that contribute to a fulfilling and balanced life. Throughout the exploration of key aspects in this comprehensive guide, including weight loss, nutrition, exercise, mindfulness, sleep, hydration, social support, and overcoming challenges, a holistic approach emerges as the cornerstone for sustainable progress.

Reflecting on the Journey:

The road to a healthier lifestyle is not a linear path but rather a continuous journey marked by progress, setbacks, and personal growth. It's crucial to recognize and celebrate every step forward, acknowledging that success is not defined solely by the destination but by the daily choices and commitment to well-being.

Key Takeaways:

1. Holistic Approach: Embracing a holistic approach that integrates physical, mental, and emotional well-being is essential. Recognizing the interconnectedness of these aspects empowers individuals to make informed choices that contribute to overall health.

2. Balanced Nutrition: The foundation of a healthy lifestyle lies in balanced nutrition. Understanding the principles of a well-rounded diet, portion control, and mindful eating fosters a sustainable relationship with food.

3. Effective Exercise Routines: Incorporating regular physical activity, tailored to individual preferences and abilities, is paramount. From simple daily movements to structured workouts, finding joy in being active contributes not only to physical health but also to mental and emotional well-being.

4. Mindful Living: Building mindfulness into everyday life, from eating habits to stress management, enhances awareness and cultivates a positive mindset. Mindfulness serves as a powerful tool in overcoming challenges and embracing a more intentional and fulfilling existence.

5. Quality Sleep and Stress Management: Prioritizing adequate sleep and effective stress management is foundational for overall health. Creating a sleep-friendly environment, practicing relaxation techniques, and addressing stressors contribute to resilience and well-being.

6. Hydration: The importance of hydration cannot be overstated. Consistent water intake supports bodily functions, aids in digestion, and contributes to energy levels. Developing habits that promote hydration is a simple yet impactful aspect of a healthy lifestyle.

7. Social Support and Accountability: Building a supportive network and fostering accountability play crucial roles in sustaining motivation and progress. Sharing goals, seeking support, and engaging with like-minded individuals create a sense of community that enhances the health journey.

8. Overcoming Challenges: Challenges are inherent in any transformative journey. The ability to navigate plateaus, setbacks, and obstacles requires resilience, adaptability, and a positive mindset. Embracing setbacks as opportunities for learning and growth fosters long-term success.

9. Celebrating Success and Maintaining Progress: Recognizing and celebrating achievements, both big and small, is a powerful motivator. Sustaining progress involves setting realistic goals, adapting to changing circumstances, and maintaining a balance between ambition and self-compassion.

10. Inspirational Stories: Drawing inspiration from real-life stories showcases the diversity of health journeys. From weight loss transformations to triumphs over emotional challenges, these narratives highlight the human capacity for resilience, determination, and positive change.

Looking Ahead:

As individuals embark on their health and well-being journeys, it's important to approach the future with a sense of curiosity, openness, and a commitment to continual growth. The guide provided here serves as a resource and framework, offering insights and practical strategies for navigating the complexities of a holistic approach to health.

Ongoing Learning and Adaptation:

The field of health and well-being is dynamic, with ongoing research, evolving perspectives, and emerging practices. Staying informed, remaining open to new information, and adapting one's approach based on individual needs contribute to sustained progress.

Community and Shared Wisdom:

The power of community and shared wisdom is evident in the collective experiences and insights shared throughout this guide. Engaging in conversations, seeking support, and learning from others create a rich tapestry of knowledge that strengthens the collective journey toward health.

Empowerment Through Choice:

Ultimately, the journey toward health is a personal and empowering experience. Every choice made in favor of well-being is a step toward a healthier, more vibrant life. Empowerment comes not only from the choices made but also from the awareness that each individual has the capacity to shape their health narrative.

A Call to Action:

In conclusion, let this guide be a call to action—a call to prioritize health, embrace positive changes, and cultivate a lifestyle that aligns with individual values and aspirations. Whether starting a new chapter or continuing an ongoing journey, remember that every decision, every effort, and every celebration contributes to the overall tapestry of well-being.

As the journey unfolds, may it be marked by resilience, joy, and a deep sense of fulfillment. Here's to the countless steps, both small and significant, that collectively form a life lived with intention, purpose, and a commitment to health.

www.ingramcontent.com/pod-product-compliance
Lightning Source LLC
Chambersburg PA
CBHW080921260726
48661CB00009B/3765